Fitness in Focus
Mindful Exercise for Lasting Wellness

Table of Contents

Chapter 1. Introduction

Welcome to an enlightening journey towards a harmonious blend of mind, body, and spirit in our Special Report, "Fitness in Focus: Mindful Exercise for Lasting Wellness." Within these pages, you'll discover the extraordinary potential of adopting mindful exercise practices not only to transform your fitness levels but also to instill an enduring sense of wellness. Painting the landscape of fitness with the vibrant hues of mindfulness, our expert guidance provides valuable insights into the joyful journey towards a healthier, happier you. Prepare to be captivated, not by grueling workouts and restrictive diets, but by a refreshing perspective that infuses loving awareness into every stretch, stride, and breath. This isn't just another fitness report; it's your passport to long-lasting holistic health. Advance towards a balanced life today; because when fitness meets mindfulness, every step becomes invigorating, every moment an opportunity to evolve!

Chapter 2. Unveiling Mindful Exercise: Demystifying the Concept

Mindfulness, to borrow the eloquent definition of Jon Kabat-Zinn, pioneer of modern mindfulness studies, represents "paying attention in a particular way; On purpose, in the present moment, and nonjudgmentally." Mindful exercise, thus, encompasses a range of activities that integrate the body-mind connection, facilitating greater awareness of oneself and the environment.

Now let's explore further:

2.1. Understanding Mindful Exercise

The essence of mindful exercise lies in its holistic approach, intertwining the realms of physical fitness and mental awareness. It seeks not just to improve physical strength, flexibility, or endurance, but also to foster a sense of connectivity and accord among body, mind, and environment.

A mindful workout employs conscious physical movement coordinated with mindful breathing, seeking to cultivate a deepening sense of presence and intentionality. This may take the form of a silent walk in the woods, a meditative yoga session, or a concentrated time spent lifting weights. What differs is the operative element of mindfulness, which dials down the blare of our frenetic lifestyles, bringing into focus the sensations of the body, the rhythm of breath, the form of movement.

2.2. Navigating the Benefits of Mindful Exercise

Mindful exercise offers a diverse array of physical, mental, and emotional benefits that stretch far beyond conventional forms of exercise. To effectively illustrate how these benefits manifest in real-life scenarios, let's use the metaphor of a tree growing in the wild.

Starting with our roots, mindful exercises like yoga, Pilates, or Tai Chi strengthens our physical foundation by improving balance, flexibility, and strength. It assists with pain management, reduces blood pressure, and enhances cardiovascular health—forming a robust 'trunk' of resilience against disease and age-related physical decline.

As branches reaching for the sky, the mental benefits of mindful exercise include enhanced cognitive functioning, improved concentration, and reduced mental fatigue. Mindful practices dovetail with exercises to enhance logical reasoning, memory recall, creative imagination, and effective problem-solving - the 'leaves' of our cognitive tree.

And finally, as fruits ripe for harvest, the emotional benefits of mindful exercise hold no less significance. It helps manage stress and reduces anxiety. It cultivates greater self-awareness, heightens empathy, nurtures positivity—fruits that sweeten our lived experience, adding richness and flavor.

2.3. The Mechanics of Mindful Exercise

An essential aspect of mindful exercise is its emphasis on form and technique over speed and repetition. This is a key departure from many conventional exercise regimes that primarily value sweat-inducing, calorie-burning activities to notch fitness goals.

The first essential is to focus on breath. Breathing is usually automatic, seemingly trivial, but it holds enormous transformative power. The breath serves as a bridge between the mind and the body. While performing an exercise, mindful breathing allows us to tune into the body's immediate responses and act accordingly.

Second, is attention to form. As we coat our physical movements with conscious attention, we start to understand the body's mechanics better. Paying attention to how the muscles contract and relax, how the body maintains balance, how the joints align during an activity, we transform our exercise from a mere series of movements to an engaging conversation with our body.

Lastly, there is the element of non-judgment. To approach exercise with a mindful lens, one must erase notions of societal definitions of success, expectations, or self-criticism. This means accepting the body as it is in the current moment, appreciating its abilities and limitations.

2.4. Applying Mindfulness During Exercise

Learning to incorporate mindfulness in your exercise routine need not be intimidating. As we've learned, the cornerstone of mindfulness rests in awareness and non-judgment. Anyone at any fitness level can begin their mindful workout journey.

Begin with straightforward tasks, such as going for a leisurely walk. However, rather than obsessing over the number of steps or the speed, focus on the sensation of your feet kissing the earth, the rhythm of your breath, the breeze on your skin, the bird's song punctuating the stillness.

Carry this idea over to your workout routine, whether it's a simple stretching or a high-intensity interval training (HIIT). Make a conscious effort to experience each stretch or each lift, the sharp intake of breath, the effort coursing through your muscles.

End by spending a few minutes in silent meditation. Allow the body to relax, the mind to rest, observing without judgment any sensations, thoughts, or feelings that may arise.

To summarize, mindful exercise represents more than a physical activity; it is a practice where moving mindfully allows us to tap into a reservoir of untapped potential, fostering not only physical fitness but also a deeper connection with our own selves and the world around us. Remember, it is not about achieving perfection, but about adopting an attitude of curiosity, acceptance, and loving-kindness towards the self. Isn't that a far healthier, harmonious, and fulfilling way toward long-lasting wellness?

Chapter 3. The Science behind Mindful Exercise: Proven Benefits for Body and Mind

The core of mindful exercise lies in consciously reconnecting the mind and body. To truly appreciate its profound impact, it's critical that we delve into the science that analytically supports its benefits.

3.1. The Integrated Functioning of the Mind and Body

The intricate symbiosis between the mind and body forms the foundation for mindful exercise. The concept of this interconnectedness dates back to ancient philosophical theories and has recently been validated through progressive fields of psychoneuroimmunology and neurobiology.

Research reveals that the body's physiological processes are significantly affected by cognitive and emotional states, heightening the importance of mental health in general well-being and fitness. Simultaneously, the state of physical health influences mood and cognition, creating a bidirectional link between the mind and body.

This dual influence is notably evidenced in the realm of stress. Prolonged stress can result in cortisol, a potentially harmful hormone, leading to a cascade of harmful physical effects ranging from heart disease to digestive problems. Conversely, physical attributes like poor nutrition and lack of exercise can exacerbate stress levels.

Seeing this, the importance of harmonizing the mind and body becomes evident, setting the stage for the concept of mindful exercise.

3.2. Neuroplasticity and Mindful Exercise

Foremost among the scientific principles related to mindful exercise is neuroplasticity – the brain's ability to restructure itself in response to experience and learning. Studies show that practicing mindfulness can change the physical structure of the brain.

Regular physical activity increases the number of neurons in the brain and strengthens their connections. High-intensity exercise prompts the release of Brain-Derived Neurotrophic Factor (BDNF), supporting the survival of existing neurons while encouraging the growth and differentiation of new neurons and synapses.

When exercise is coupled with mindfulness, the brain benefits manifold. Practicing mindful exercise stimulates the prefrontal cortex – responsible for executive functions such as decision-making and social behavior – and decreases the activity of the amygdala, associated with fear and stress. This change ultimately amplifies the positive neuroplastic changes induced by exercise alone.

3.3. Biomarkers and Mindful Exercise

A range of biomarkers correlates exercise and stress levels with physical health. Cortisol levels, for instance, rise in response to stress. Chronic high cortisol can lead to a series of health issues, ranging from obesity and diabetes, to mental health conditions.

Research has substantiated that mindful exercise leads to a drop in cortisol levels. For example, a study conducted on individuals who practiced mindful yoga found a significant decrease in cortisol and perceived stress levels, while simultaneously observing an increase in immune markers.

Another such biomarker is Interleukin-6 (IL-6), a pro-inflammatory cytokine that plays a vital role in fighting infection and healing injuries. However, chronic elevation in IL-6 levels is linked to several inflammatory diseases. Mindful exercises such as Tai Chi have been found to lower IL-6 levels considerably.

3.4. Cardiometabolic Health and Mindful Exercise

Mindful exercises have profound effects on cardiometabolic health. Regular physical activity strengthens the heart muscle, amplifies lung capacity, and boosts metabolism, contributing to overall fitness and weight management.

Observational studies show that when mindfulness is combined with exercise, one is likely to stick to a physical activity regimen better, thereby reaping the sustained longer-term benefits of physical activity on the reduction of cardiovascular risk factors.

3.5. Mental Health and Mindful Exercise

Mindful exercise can have a profound impact on mental health. Mindful exercise helping in managing depression, reducing anxiety, and improving mood and sleep quality, are well-accepted within the psychological and psychiatric communities.

Mindful exercise has been shown to activate the parasympathetic nervous system, which calms the body and counteracts the fight-orflight response related to stress. As a result, it can serve as a non-pharmaceutical tool to manage different mental health disorders.

3.6. Longevity and Mindful Exercise

The combination of mindfulness and exercise may potentially influence longevity. Telomeres, the protective caps at the end of chromosomes, tend to shorten as cells divide and age. High levels of psychological stress are associated with shorter telomeres, thus faster cellular aging.

Practices combining mindfulness and exercise (like Yoga and Tai Chi) have been found to positively affect telomere length, suggesting that they might have various anti-aging effects.

3.7. The Defining Verdict

In conclusion, from neurobiology to cardiology, from endocrinology to psychology, science substantiates the tremendous potential of mindful exercise. The fusion of mindfulness with physical activity harnesses a far-reaching array of benefits that span the spectrum of human health. By integrating the mind and body via exercise, we unlock a deeper level of awareness, preparation, and resilience, guiding us into a fulfilled existence. Mindful exercise is not just a fitness trend; it's a revolution in human health and wellbeing. It's a call for us to be completely present and harmonize every aspect of our being. It's a way to not just live, but thrive.

Chapter 4. Decoding Mindfulness: The Art of Living in the Present

Attention research indicates that our minds wander almost half the time. Whether contemplating yesterday's regrets, tomorrow's to-dos, or any fleeting thought, we miss the richness of now, the only reality we truly inhabit. In this context emerges mindfulness - the art of living in the present.

4.1. The Elixir of Mindfulness

The term 'mindfulness' is a translation of the Pali word 'sati', a significant element of Buddhist tradition. Yet, it transcends cultural and religious boundaries. We map its nuances by defining it as a process of maintaining a moment-by-moment awareness of our thoughts, feelings, sensations, and the surrounding environment, through a gentle, nurturing lens.

Jon Kabat-Zinn, a pioneering authority on mindfulness, defines it as "paying attention in a particular way, on purpose, in the present moment, and non-judgmentally." It invites us to wake up from our mechanical, conditioning-ridden life, to step off the hamster wheel of habitual reactions, and to start experiencing the grandeur of being right here, right now.

4.2. Anchoring in the Present

A mindful state does not magically occur; it takes sincere practice. Notice the urge to rush through the day, leaping from one task to another. Begin by slowing down, fully immersing in the current activity, whether eating, walking, or even breathing.

One simple, accessible form of mindfulness practice is meditation. Sit in a quiet place, close your eyes, take a deep breath, slowly release it and repeat. Wordlessly observe each breath, inhalation and exhalation, without trying to control or judge it. If your mind begins to wander, and it will, gently draw it back to the breath.

A basic mindful walking practice involves focusing on the sensation of your feet touching the ground. The key is not to consider the destination as the goal, but to pay attention to each step, commit to the journey.

4.3. Distilling Benefits from Mindfulness

The range of benefits offered by mindfulness appear almost magical yet are scientifically backed. Enhancements in mental health, emotional stability, sleep quality, and even physical health are just a few to start with.

Mindfulness reduces stress by breaking down our experiences into smaller parts, dismantling overwhelming tasks or bouts of anxiety. It offers us a safe harbor, an oasis of calm amidst the storm of life's challenges.

Research reveals that mindfulness-developed self-compassion helps combat depression. By gently welcoming and accepting our darker shades, mindfulness helps us cultivate the courage to face life's adversities.

On the physical health front, mindfulness has proven effective in pain management, especially chronic pain, by altering the perception of pain and reducing rumination. It's also beneficial for gastrointestinal disorders and improves heart health.

4.4. Mindful Fitness: An Integrated Approach

The amplification of fitness through mindfulness lies in not just doing a particular exercise, but in immersing yourself fully in the experience. It shifts the focus from striving for a perfect body to cultivating a loving acceptance of your body, encouraging its nurturing through enjoyable exercises.

Mind-body exercises such as yoga, Tai Chi, and Qigong are great for building mindfulness and fitness together. These practices engage the mind and the body, fostering an increased sense of body awareness, improving balance and flexibility, and enhancing breathing.

Next time you lift weights, run, or cycle, pay attention to each movement, to the sensation in your muscles. Feel the ground as you jog, the air as it brushes past you, the rhythm of your breath – these are your connections to the present, to life itself.

4.5. Keep Growing, Keep Evolving

Mindfulness, like physical fitness, is not a goal one can complete or a destination one can reach. They are daily practices, moments of connection. It's a continuous, personal journey towards self-discovery, growth, and an integrated wellness approach.

It's about fully opening up to life as it unfolds moment by moment, not getting lost in 'shoulds' and 'musts' of future achievements or past disappointments. This doesn't mean we discard the past or future; we merely accord the present its rightful priority.

Through the rhythmic dance of mindfulness and fitness, we can learn to navigate life with grace, courage, and joy. So, tune into the grand symphony of life playing out right here, right now because that is where the magic happens.

In conclusion, mindfulness, as an art and skill, offers a transformative journey towards living in the present. It cultivates a deeper, more enriching relationship with our own bodies and minds. It's the golden thread weaving our experiences, seamlessly integrating mind, body, and spirit, ensuring our journey towards holistic wellness is promising, enjoyable, and fulfilling.

Chapter 5. Getting Started: Essential Mindful Exercises for Beginners

The first step in delving into the world of mindful exercise is understanding it. The concept of being physically present, focusing both attention and awareness on the task at hand, is as simple as it is profound. Whether you're a seasoned athlete, a complete beginner, or somewhere in between, you can start benefitting from mindful exercises today.

5.1. The Power of Breath

Our journey starts where we all do - with breath. Breathing seems as simple as being alive, but correct, mindful breathing is fundamental to our health and well-being . Right here, right now, let's get started.

1. Sit in a neutral position, creating a strong yet comfortable base. Sit on the front edge of a comfortable chair with your feet flat on the floor, or perhaps cross-legged on a yoga mat or cushion.

2. Start by observing your natural breath. In times of rest, our breath is often shallow and centered in the chest. For now, just observe.

3. Now, let's consciously alter our breathing. Inhale deeply through your nose, feeling your belly rise as it fills with air.

4. Exhale slowly through the mouth, considerably slower than the inhale. Feel your belly fall.

5. Repeat this patterned breathing for about five minutes.

This exercise is a basic introduction to focused, conscious breathing which in itself is a form of mindfulness practice. It prepares the body for more active exercises soon to come, facilitating a state of mind that supports deeper connection with your body, feelings, and present moment.

5.2. Yoga and Mindfulness

A dynamic blend of mindfulness and physical exercise, yoga is a quintessential mindful exercise. For beginners, though, yoga can seem inaccessible or intimidating, with talk of impossible-looking poses and spiritual detachment. Fear not. Yoga is about progression, not perfection.

5.3. Start with the Mountain Pose

Simplicity is the beauty of the Mountain Pose or Tadasana, a foundation pose for many others. Here's how to do it:

1. Stand tall with your feet hip-width apart, toes pointing forward.

2. Spread your toes wide and distribute your weight evenly across both feet to anchor strongly.

3. Pull up your kneecaps subtly, and engage your thigh muscles. Tilt your pelvis slightly forward.

4. Inhale, and lift your chest, standing up tall and straight but relaxed.

5. Exhale and drop your shoulders away from your ears, allowing tension to exit your body.

6. Reach your fingertips down towards the floor, arms relaxed by your side. Imagine you're stretching towards the earth.

7. Breathe deeply for several breaths, maintaining your attention on the pose.

5.4. Progress to Warrior I Pose

Building from the Mountain Pose, the Warrior I Pose, or Virabhadrasana I, is more active and engaging. How to proceed:

1. Start in Mountain Pose, then step your right foot back about one leg's length.

2. Turn your right foot 45 degrees outward. Ensure your left foot points forward.

3. Bend your left knee till it's directly above the ankle, forming a right angle. Keep your right leg straight.

4. Inhale and sweep your arms out to the sides and up toward the sky, lifting your chest. Keep your gaze forward or up towards your hands, depending on your neck comfort.

5. Hold for several breaths, keeping your mind attuned to the stretch in your legs and the reaching of your hands. Repeat on the other side.

Yoga is often associated with flexibility, but it's not just about flexibility of body. It's about flexibility of mind - a willingness to try, to persevere, and to adapt. So breathe, stretch, and appreciate what you accomplish along the way.

5.5. Moving Meditation: The Power of Walking

Not every mindful exercise requires a yoga mat or special gear. Walking, an activity that we all engage in everyday, can be transformed into a mindfulness practice. Here's a simple way to transform a regular walk into mindful walking:

1. Begin walking at a slow pace, in a safe and quiet space.

2. With every step, pay attention to the lifting and falling of your

foot as it makes contact with the ground.

3. Observe the weight transfer across your foot, from heel to toe.

4. Focus your attention on your breath, body, and the sensations of each step.

5. When your mind starts to wander, gently bring it back to the sensations of walking.

For most of us, walking is a means to an end - to get from one place to another. By contrast, mindful walking is a journey in itself. Shift away from the objective, and focus on the process. This simple mindful exercise can be wonderfully grounding and calming.

5.6. The Importance of Regular Practice

Patience and consistency are key when adopting mindful exercises. Like any skill, practice makes perfect. Remember, this is not a contest, but a personal journey. Every small step you make brings you closer to a healthier, happier self.

In the end, mindfulness in exercise is about honoring the deep connection between mind and body. Our bodies are beautiful, complex systems that do so much for us; they deserve our respect and appreciation. So, no matter how your journey in mindful exercise begins, always be patient, be kind, and allow yourself to enjoy the process. Fitness is a journey, not a destination.

Chapter 6. Yoga and Mindfulness: A Dynamic Duo for Wholesome Wellness

The intertwined relationship of Yoga and Mindfulness curates a wholesome wellness path, offering treasures of enhanced mental clarity, physical vitality, and emotional stability. The duo's unique synergistic nature can reboot your wellness journey, guiding you towards living a balanced, mindful, and healthy life.

6.1. The Communion of Yoga and Mindfulness

Yoga, a science that dates back thousands of years, holds the transformative power to harmonize the body, mind, and spirit. When combined with Mindfulness—a simple, powerful practice focusing all awareness on the present moment — the outcome is a potent concoction that deeply influences both physical wellness and inner equilibrium.

Yoga, at its heart, is more than just a collection of physical poses. It is a rich philosophical system that encourages us to find peace and balance amidst life's chaos. Mindfulness too, empowers individuals to align themselves with the present, thereby fostering an attitude of acceptance and providing an antidote to the strain of modern life. When combined, Yoga and Mindfulness seize the power to lead us towards a more conscious existence filled with health and harmony.

6.2. Unraveling the Benefits: Body, Mind, and Spirit

The fusion of Yoga and Mindfulness offers significantly more than the sum of their individual benefits. This powerful blend exercises our body, harmonizes our spirit, and calms our mind, helping us dive deeper into the essence of our being.

6.2.1. Physical Strengthening and Flexibility

Regular yoga practice enhances muscle strength, augments flexibility and boosts endurance. Yoga asanas, or postures, are designed to work on different parts of the body, from the spinal cord to the joints to the muscles, focusing on every element to achieve a diverse range of motions. By incorporating this routine systematically and progressively, one can gradually build up physical strength and resilience. Coupling it with mindful breathing and movements makes the practice even more potent, nurturing a deep sense of connection with the physical self.

6.2.2. Mental Equilibrium and Clarity

Mindfulness exercises – best personified in mindful meditation – can lead to reduced stress levels, a serene state of mind, and improved cognitive abilities. When combined with Yoga, which promotes similar benefits, the result is amplified mental wellness. Concentrating on the here and now during a Yoga session forces the mind to let go of past regrets and future worries. This mindful practice cultivates an enhanced state of mental welness and clarity.

6.2.3. Enhanced Emotional Stability

Regular practice of Yoga and mindfulness helps in managing negative emotions, improving mood, and nurturing inner peace. Being fully present and aware during Yoga practice allows for better understanding of various complex emotions that rise to the surface. This increased understanding helps in managing emotional responses more effectively and fosters emotional stability.

6.3. Incorporating Yoga and Mindfulness into Everyday Life

Achieving holistic wellness through Yoga and Mindfulness goes beyond intermittent practices or sessions. It comprises of integrating these principles into everyday life.

6.3.1. Setting an Intention

Before you start with your Yoga practice, setting an intention can be transformative. This intention, or 'Sankalpa' in Yoga, could be a short positive statement or simply a word that resonates with what you seek from the practice. It not only sets the tone for your routine, but its constant repetition can channelize your subconscious mind towards achieving the intended goal.

6.3.2. Cultivating Presence

Incorporating mindfulness into Yoga means to be fully present during the practice. It entails focusing on the asanas, observing your breath and body, and perceiving every sensation. It's about detaching from external distractions and delving deeper into oneself.

6.3.3. Mindful Eating and Living

Bringing mindfulness to eating can enhance your relationship with food, thereby promoting physical health and overall wellness. Noticing the texture, taste and aroma of what you're eating slows down the process, aiding digestion, preventing overeating and increasing diet satisfaction. Beyond eating, mindfulness when incorporated into daily activities like walking, working or even taking a shower, amplifies awareness and brings an enriched sense of being.

6.4. A Journey, Not a Destination

It's crucial to remember that the confluence of Yoga and Mindfulness is a lifelong journey. Every day offers unique challenges and experiences that test our resolve and core. By remembering to be kind to ourselves, acknowledging that progress is not linear, and treating each moment as a new opportunity to grow – we can rightfully embrace the dynamic duo's journey towards wholesome wellness.

In conclusion, the blend of Yoga and Mindfulness acts as a powerhouse, paving the way to a healthier and happier life. By effectively managing stress, strengthening the body, and improving emotional stability, it certainly makes a compelling case for a lifestyle choice worth considering.

Mindful exercise is not just about changing your body; it's about changing your life. So, leverage this dynamic duo and embark on this glorious journey towards lasting wellness. Today, you're just a few mindful breaths and stretch away from a healthier, happier you. So, take that first step. Unleash the extraordinary potential of Yoga and Mindfulness. Remember, it's never too late to start.

Remember, the best time to begin is now. Following the path the dynamic duo lays out, you will find yourself becoming more alive, more in-tune, and more aware, not just on the Yoga mat, but in the grand stage of life itself. You are on the verge of commencing a journey into a territory filled with profound experiences, stronger health, and pure joy. So dive in. The magic of Yoga and mindfulness awaits.

Chapter 7. Guided Mindful Running: Fitness with Awareness

Before we venture into the specifics of mindful running, it's important to set a solid groundwork. Understanding the foundation of mindful running helps you harness your full potential. Keep in mind that mindful running doesn't follow a one-size-fits-all routine; it's about your connection with your own body, mind, and environment.

As you embark on this fulfilling journey, bear in mind that this isn't about replacing your existing running practice but rather about enriching it. The beauty of mindful running resides in its flexibility to be adopted and adapted to any running schedule.

7.1. The Philosophy of Mindful Running

Before we lace up our running shoes, let's begin by sketching a picture of the concept, philosophy, and benefits of mindful running. Mindful running combines the physical act of running with the awareness-based practice of mindfulness. It's about engaging fully in the present moment, paying attention to the sensations in your body, your surroundings, and the rhythm of your breath as you move.

By integrating mindfulness into running, we can not only improve our physical performance through better focus but also garner numerous mental and emotional benefits such as reduced stress, increased mental clarity, and enhanced mood. It's a holistic practice that targets not just physical fitness, but mental and emotional wellbeing as well.

7.2. Tuning into Physical Sensations

Start by focusing on your body. As you run, tune into the sensations from each part of your body - from the rhythmic bounce in your steps, the stretching of your muscles, the swinging of your arms, to the gentle inhale and exhale of your breath. Observing these sensations cultivates an intimate relationship with your body, making you more in tune with your physical self.

7.3. Sensing the Surrounding Environment

By paying attention to the environment around you as you run, you become more connected to the world. Feel the wind on your skin, listen to the ambient sounds, notice the colors and movements of the landscape. This mindful observation not only enhances your environmental awareness but also fosters a profound sense of connectedness with nature.

7.4. The Power of Breath in Mindful Running

Breath is an important and often overlooked aspect of running. By concentrating on your breath - its rhythm, depth, and pace - you can manage your running cadence better. Additionally, focusing on your breath helps reduce mental chatter, providing a quiet space for reflection as your feet kiss the pavement.

7.5. Starting Your Mindful Running Practice

To begin your mindful running journey, start with shorter runs, using them as a kind of moving meditation. Initially, it will be tempting to slip back into your normal running mode, but stay patient with yourself. It is a practice, after all, and it will take time to foster this new habit.

7.6. Setting the Pace

Starting off too hard and too fast is a common mistake in running. In mindful running, you set your pace, remembering that this is not a race. Your aim isn't just covering distance or increasing speed, but rather running with awareness, attention, and presence.

7.7. Body Scan Meditations

Start your run with a body scan meditation, checking in with each part of your body. This will help center your mind, heighten bodily awareness, and prepare you for your mindful run.

7.8. Breathing Techniques

Experiment with various breathing techniques to find what suits you. Some enjoy counting breaths, while others prefer syncing their breath with their steps. You may find it useful to start with deep, slow breaths to calm your nervous system before picking up the pace.

7.9. Mindful Running Drills

Integrate various mindful running drills into your workout to make it more engaging and functional. These might include focusing on a single body part, tuning in to your natural surroundings, or chanting a mindful mantra.

7.10. The Challenges of Mindful Running

Mindful running, like any new habit, comes with its own set of challenges. At first, you may face difficulties concentrating or staying in the moment. Recognize these as part of your growth and not as failures. Give yourself room to learn and adapt.

7.11. Cultivating a Regular Practice

Over time, as mindful running becomes a more natural part of your running routine, you may find that your runs are more enjoyable, fulfilling, and less injury-prone. This will buoy you to cultivate it as a regular practice.

The path of mindful running is the path of connecting - to your body, to your environment, and most importantly, to the present moment. This art of combining mindfulness and running can transform your physical workouts into an enriching mental and spiritual experience. So, lace up those shoes, step out with an open mind, and allow mindful running to guide your journey towards lasting wellness.

Chapter 8. Mindful Strength Training: An Unexplored Arena

Traditionally, strength training has been an area largely dominated by the physical aspects of health, with minimal attention paid to the psychological or emotional effects. However, the concept of Mindful Strength Training pushes this boundary and invites us to integrate mindfulness into our strength training routine.

8.1. The Fusion of Mindfulness and Strength Training

Strength training has often been thought of as focusing solely on the body. You lift a weight, and it makes your muscles grow, right? But what if we were to add another layer to this? What if we were to introduce the principles of mindfulness into this process?

Let's begin by looking at the concept of mindfulness. This is a mental state achieved by focusing one's awareness on the present moment, calmly acknowledging and accepting one's feelings, thoughts, and bodily sensations. Imagine bringing this level of mindfulness into your strength training. You would not just be lifting weights; you would be experiencing the sensations, appreciating your body's resilience, and valuing every moment of the journey. This powerful blend infuses every workout with a deeper sense of purpose and connection.

At its core, Mindful Strength Training represents the ideal blend of mental and physical fitness - it is fitness in its most holistic sense. By fusing mindfulness with strength training, we can create a workout routine that amplifies the benefits of both these practices.

8.2. The Practice of Mindful Strength Training

The process of integrating mindfulness and strength training begins by focusing on the 'mind' in mind-body connection. It's about bringing your full presence to every rep, immersing yourself fully in the process, and experiencing everything your body goes through.

Start with a warm-up routine. As you stretch, notice the sensation in your muscles, the rhythm of your breath, how your body feels. Once you begin lifting weights, draw your attention to the muscles contracting and relaxing. Be aware of your posture, your grip on the weight, and how your body moves. With every rep, notice how your muscles respond, the warmth permeating through them, the sense of accomplishment with each completed set.

Breathing plays a pivotal role in Mindful Strength Training. Each inhalation brings energy, while every exhalation releases fatigue. As you lift, exhale, and as you lower the weight, inhale. This not only enhances performance but solidifies the mind-body connection.

8.3. Benefits of Mindful Strength Training

Mindful Strength Training is highly beneficial, impacting every aspect of our fitness journey.

- Improved Awareness: By being present in the here and now, mindful strength training enhances your overall sense of body awareness. This is vital, as it helps you maintain correct body mechanics, ensures effective targeting of muscle groups, and ultimately leads to optimal workout results.

- Increased Focus: The practice of mindful strength training helps develop an intense level of concentration. This translates into better performance in the workout routine, resulting in accelerated fitness gains.

- Stress Reduction: Working synergistically, mindfulness and strength training help mitigate stress and anxiety levels. The endorphins released during strength training, combined with the calming effects of mindfulness, provide a potent stress-relieving combination.

- Enhanced Emotional Health: Through a regular mindful strength training regimen, we can cultivate emotional stability, bolster self-esteem, and foster a sense of accomplishment.

8.4. Mindful Strength Training: A Practical How-to Guide

The following are some practical tips to integrate mindfulness into your strength training routine:

- Start with a purpose: Before you begin, set an intention for your workout. It could be to build strength, resilience, mindfulness, or simply to feel good.

- Feel the weight: As you grip your weight, be mindful of the feel. Is it cold? Heavy? Rough? Allow your attention to register this sensation.

- Be Present: As you do your reps, don't just go through the motion. Be present. Feel each muscle contraction, the stretch, the fatigue, the rest.

- Breathe Mindfully: Be aware of your breathing. Let the rhythm of your breath match your workout. Inhale deeply when you lift, exhale as you lower.

- Celebrate: Each completed set is a milestone, a testament to your persistence. Value the feeling of accomplishment. Savor it before moving on.

Each of these steps, when combined and practiced regularly, can lead to substantial improvements, both physically and mentally. This approach enables individuals to experience a deeper involvement with their bodies and the workout process, leading to a fitness regimen that delivers multidimensional benefits.

In conclusion, today, as we endeavor to lead healthier and more fulfilled lives, the paradigm of fitness is shifting from simply 'looking good' to 'feeling good', from rapid transformations to sustainable changes. Mindful Strength Training represents this evolution in fitness. It is an unexplored arena teeming with potential, offering an incredibly promising pathway to personal growth and wellness. With its emphasis on balance, self-awareness, and inner harmony, it's not merely an exercise regime - it's a way of life.

With conscious effort and continual practice, anyone can master mindful strength training. Unleash your potential and make exercise a meditative process - a harmonious symphony where body, mind, and soul perform together, celebrating their combined strength and resilience. It's time we recognized the power of holistic health and accessed the extraordinary potential within all of us. Whether you are a seasoned athlete, fitness enthusiast, or starting your journey, Mindful Strength Training may just be the transformative practice you've been seeking.

Chapter 9. Embodying Mindfulness: Nutritional Choices for Mind-Body Harmony

Learning to feed your mind, body, and spirit with mindful nutrition is a crucial step in harmonizing the health of each. Here, we explore the application of mindfulness principles to your daily nutritional choices, bringing forth the concept of eating mindfully, respectfully, and with an utter understanding of our bodies' needs and responses to food.

9.1. Understanding Mindful Eating

Mindful eating is a practice that draws on the principles of mindfulness, encouraging us to slow down, pay attention to the food we consume, and experience the sensations of eating fully. It involves recognizing and respecting our body's needs, distinguishing between physical hunger and emotional hunger, and developing an understanding of how our food choices impact our health and well-being.

Mindful eating is not about restriction or depriving ourselves. Instead, it's about truly savoring our food, being present during meals, and listening to what our bodies tell us about our needs and satisfaction levels.

9.2. The Role of Mindfulness in Making Nutritional Choices

Mindfulness is the act of paying attention on purpose, in the present moment, and nonjudgmentally. When applied to eating, it involves paying attention to our food and our body's responses to food without judgment.

Through mindfulness, we can learn to recognize our body's signals about hunger and satiety. We can make more conscious nutritional choices, avoiding mindless eating habits like eating out of boredom, stress, or habit. Mindful eaters tend to choose foods that are more nourishing and satisfying, leading to improved health and a more balanced diet.

9.3. The Path to Mindful Eating

This shift to mindful eating is a journey that takes time and practice. It starts with paying attention to the food you eat, appreciating the flavors, the texture, the color, and smell. Here are steps you can take on your path to mindful eating:

1. Pause before you eat: Take a moment to appreciate the food in front of you. Notice the colors, smells, and textures. Acknowledge the effort taken to prepare the meal.

2. Eat slowly: Put your utensils down between bites. Chew slowly and thoroughly before swallowing to truly taste the flavors of the food.

3. Pay attention to hunger and fullness cues: Learn to recognize your body's signals. Stop eating when you feel satisfied, not when you have cleaned your plate.

4. Reduce distractions: Turn off the TV, put away your phone, and make meals a time for connection and enjoyment, not

multitasking.

5. Experiment with food: Try new foods and flavors to keep your meals interesting and enjoyable.

9.4. The Nutritional Side: A Mindful Plate

Including a variety of wholesome, nutrient-dense foods in your diet is the key to fueling your body properly. A mindful plate can include fruits, vegetables, lean proteins, healthy fats, and whole grains.

Here is an example of what a mindful plate could look like:

- Half your plate filled with colorful vegetables: Each color represents different nutrients, so a variety is key.

- A quarter of your plate dedicated to lean proteins: This could be from animal or plant sources.

- A quarter of your plate for whole grains: Opt for grains like brown rice, quinoa, or oats.

- Include healthy fats: Add a handful of nuts, seeds, or avocado to your meal for some beneficial fats.

9.5. Cultivating a Mindful Relationship with Food

It's important to remember that mindful eating is not just a diet or a weight-loss strategy: it is a practice of awareness. We can use it as a tool to cultivate a healthier, more balanced relationship with food that transcends meal times.

- Mindful grocery shopping: Look at the food labels, understand the ingredients, source fresh and whole foods whenever possible.

- Mindful cooking: Engage yourself in the process of preparing your meal; the smells, the sights and the sounds of sizzling can be quite rewarding.

- Mindful indulgence: If you crave something, enjoy it mindfully, without guilt, but in moderation.

Through mindful eating, we can discover a new relationship with food—one of respect, appreciation, and balance. We learn to honor our body's needs, nurture our health, and enjoy the intrinsic pleasures of eating. Endlessly rewarding, mindful eating is a journey that bridges the gap between mind and body, fortifying the bond that leads to enduring wellness.

The art of mindful eating, combined with sound nutritional choices, ensures that every morsel you consume adds value to your well-being, without sacrificing the joy of eating. As you harmoniously unite your mind, body, and spirit, your nutritional choices become not just a route to physical health, but a journey towards total wellness.

In conclusion, embodying mindfulness in your dietary choices enhances your overall health, inspiring balance, vitality, and longevity. It aligns your nutritional habits with self-awareness, conscious decision-making, and an open heart towards self-care. It's not just about food; it's about a balanced life filled with joy, awareness, respect, and gratitude for our body's needs and desires. Now that's a delicious and mindful way to live!

Chapter 10. Overcoming Hurdles: Strategies to Stay Committed to Your Mindful Exercise Routine

Finding commitment and motivation to stick to an exercise routine can be challenging. Driven by this understanding, we delve into the complexities of maintaining a mindful exercise routine, introducing strategies, and sharing insights that can aid your journey in overcoming hurdles and staying devoted to your plan.

10.1. Understanding the Mind-Body Connection

The mind-body connection refers to how your thoughts, feelings, and behaviors can influence your physical state. A positive mindset can foster beneficial results, while negative thinking or stress can disrupt your wellbeing.

Regular exercise has been shown to help mitigate stress and enhance overall mood, moreover, when performed mindfully, it can forge an even stronger mind-body connection.

10.2. The Role of Motivation

Motivation is the driving force behind why we act. It arises from within (intrinsic motivation) or stems from external factors (extrinsic motivation). In understanding our motivation, we can create a plan that effectively encourages consistent routine execution.

Intrinsic motivation involves engaging in an activity for personal enjoyment and self-satisfaction. Meanwhile, extrinsic motivation includes external rewards or approvals such as compliments or societal recognition.

To foster a sustainable, long-term fit lifestyle, it's imperative to cultivate a strong intrinsic motivation source. The joy of movement, feeling more energetic, or enhanced self-awareness are compelling reasons to exercise that don't rely on external validation.

10.3. The Art of Setting Goals

Success in mindful fitness begins with setting clear, achievable goals. Your goals should be SMART: Specific, Measurable, Achievable, Relevant, and Time-Bound.

Adopting SMART goals can keep you guided and focused. It also presents an opportunity to celebrate small victories along the way, boosting your motivation.

Steer away from shallow, aesthetics-driven goals. Instead, opt for targets that promote holistic health, amplify self-awareness and truly enrich your mind-body connection.

10.4. Utilizing Visualization Techniques

Visualization is a powerful tool that leverages the mind-body connection for your benefit. Regularly visualizing yourself meeting your goals can improve self-confidence and enhance motivation. It trains your mind to see the possibilities and attune your consciousness towards achieving your goal.

10.5. Maintaining a Yoga and Meditation Routine

Practices like yoga and meditation can enhance your mindfulness during exercise. Yoga strengthens the body while promoting flexibility and balance. Simultaneously, it requires mindfulness to focus on your movement and breath, helping you create a stronger connection with your body. Meditation, on the other hand, can help manage stress, enabling clearer thought processes for maintaining your exercise routine.

Encouragingly, both yoga and meditation require minimal equipment and can be practiced virtually anywhere.

10.6. Embracing the Challenges

Establishing and maintaining an exercise routine is rarely straightforward. You will face some hurdles along the way; these obstacles are part of the journey rather than setbacks. Instead of being disheartened by them, interpret them as opportunities to grow and evolve.

10.7. Managing Setbacks

Circumstances can disrupt your routine. Illness, injury, or unforeseen events can upset progress. In such instances, be gentle with yourself. Acknowledge the setback, and then determine how you can move forward without imposing unnecessary stress.

10.8. Enlisting Social Support

People around you – friends, family, or fellow athletes – can motivate you and potentially influence your adherence to your routine. By surrounding yourself with supportive individuals, you can help foster a positive environment that encourages your efforts and allows you to share your achievements and failures. If possible, consider joining a group class or finding a mindful exercise partner.

10.9. Celebrating Progress

Rewarding your progress, both big and small, can keep your motivation levels high. This doesn't always mean 'treat meals'; it can be about taking time for self-appreciation, sharing achievements with loved ones, or investing in new workout gear.

10.10. Prioritizing Self-Love and Self-Care

Remember, the journey of mindful fitness is about creating a loving relationship with your body, not punishing it. Self-love and self-care should be at the core of all your endeavors. Listen to your body, respect its needs, and offer it rest when needed.

Keeping these strategies in mind, overcoming hurdles, and staying committed to your mindful exercise routine can be far more achievable. So, embark on this journey today, and watch every stretch, every breath lead you towards a healthier, happier self.

Chapter 11. Beyond Fitness: Moving towards Holistic Wellness with Mindful Exercise

Mindful exercise is no longer a fringe element hovering on the outskirts of mainstream fitness. It has moved front and center, applauded by health professionals, exercise scientists, and neuropsychologists for its holistic approach to well-being that extends well beyond physical fitness alone. This chapter will delve into a comprehensive exploration of how mindful exercise contributes to holistic wellness, casting a broader and more profound health and fitness net.

11.1. Advantages of Incorporating Mindfulness into Exercise

Mindfulness can be understood as the state of being fully conscious or aware in the present moment. It forms the union between the mind and body, enabling them to work in harmony. When applied to exercise, mindfulness takes the focus away from the more common "no pain, no gain" approach, bringing about a host of physical and psychological benefits.

1. Improved focus and mental clarity: Moving mindfully helps you cultivate an enhanced sense of focus and attentiveness. This skill translates well beyond your workout routine and can lead to improved work performance and concentration in tasks.

2. Enhanced enjoyment: The practice of mindfulness promotes an attitude of appreciation, transforming what is often seen as a chore into an enjoyable moment-to-moment experience.

3. Stress reduction: Mindful exercise has been shown to reduce levels of stress and anxiety. The mindfulness aspect helps you tap into a profound sense of calm within the storm, allowing for better stress management.

4. Injury prevention: Mindful movements make you more attuned to your body's signals, reducing the likelihood of injury. Paying detailed attention to each movement increases your body awareness, leading you to make healthier decisions.

11.2. Mindful Exercise: Where to Begin

Getting started with mindful exercise doesn't necessitate a complete overhaul of your current fitness regimen. It only requires the introduction of an element of mindfulness. The following steps are suggested to incorporate mindfulness into your exercise routine:

1. Start with a ritual: Begin your workout with a mindfulness meditation to set the tone for your session. This could be a moment of focused breathing, an intention-setting mantra, or even a warm-up stretch performed with conscious attention.

2. Choose movements that you enjoy: You're more likely to stay present during exercises that you find enjoyable. Whether it's yoga, running, lifting weights, or dance, your exercise mode can be a powerful ally in encouraging mindfulness.

3. Focus on the quality of movement: Rather than counting repetitions or clocking the miles, focus on the quality of each movement. Notice the way your muscles engage and release, the rhythm of your breath, and how your body feels in each phase of movement.

4. Cultivate a compassionate attitude towards your body: Adopt a kinder, gentler approach towards your body. Instead of pushing obsessively towards certain targets, allow your body the space it

needs to rest and replenish.

5. Stay in the present: Don't rush through your workouts. Be fully engaged with each moment, paying careful attention to your body's signals and needs.

11.3. Applications of Mindful Exercise

Several exercise types lend themselves naturally to mindfulness. The following activities are perfect for integrating mindfulness and exercise:

1. Yoga: Yoga is a practice that inherently combines movement and mindfulness. Every position calls for deliberate engagement of muscles, balance, and breathing. It holds a mirror up to our physical and mental processes, making it a perfect mindful exercise.

2. Tai Chi: This ancient Chinese practice, often described as meditation in movement, cultivates balance, flexibility, and cardiovascular fitness. It promotes mindfulness through a series of fluid, gentle movements that flow from one into the next.

3. Walking: A simple walk can transform into a mindful exercise by focusing on the sensation of your feet hitting the ground, the rhythm of your breath, or the wind against your skin.

4. Swimming: The repetitive act of swimming can serve as a meditation. The sound of the water, the rhythm of your strokes, and your breath all contribute to a mindful experience.

5. Body-weight training: Simple bodyweight exercises such as squats, lunges, or push-ups can be done mindfully. By focusing on the quality of movements and breath, this training approach can help to improve concentration and body awareness.

Mindful exercise serves as a key to unlock an extraordinary realm where fitness is not just about losing weight or building muscles, but also about cultivating a healthier relationship with your own body. It paves the way for an enriching journey towards holistic wellness that celebrates every step, appreciating each sweat drop as an offering of love to your body. Embrace mindful exercise not merely as another aspect of your fitness routine but as a transformative lifestyle practice and embark on a beautifully harmonious journey of mind, body, and spirit.